SURVIVING
IN AN
EVER-CHANGING
HEALTHCARE
INDUSTRY

I0455083

DONNA GAULT

outskirts
press

Acknowledgments

I want to tell you first: I am not a writer. I am a nurse. I didn't write this book to dwell on the negatives, but to help. I have always been a sincere advocate for my patients and that is the motive behind this book.

My thanks go to all who not only supported me, but who added to this book. Special thanks go to two great doctors; one is a practicing hospitalist, and the other an experienced family physician. They wrote valued information in my book. I can't thank them enough for taking the time from their busy schedules to share their expertise. My sincere thanks also go to those who were willing to share their own experiences in the book.

Everyone should appreciate and thank all those who serve in the medical field. I believe this book will be especially understood by those individuals because they live it every day and most still do their very best to serve and protect everyone. They are today's medical heroes but so few are ever recognized. They don't do it to be recognized. They know it's their job. Seldom does one know the great efforts they may have gone through. They are good people, with great ethics, and truly believe it's the right thing to do. They care! I ask that God be with them on this sometimes very difficult journey.

I dedicate this book to my wonderful family, who I truly love, and especially my grandchildren, who always bring true joy to my heart.

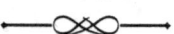

Table of Contents

Table of Contents

CHAPTER 1

A Nurse's Concerns

I started this book on December 29, 2010. At first it began with some of my personal nursing stories; then, as I wrote, I knew in my heart, it needed to be about much more. I felt the nurse advocate in me. My goal for this book was to provide information on the changes in an evolving healthcare industry, to show that right now it is a healthcare industry that could be a potential danger to families. I was hoping to help everyone survive in it.

I am an old nurse. I graduated in 1965 from a Catholic three-year diploma school in Dayton, Ohio, St. Elizabeth School of Nursing.

It was a wonderful school. Great nurses were produced. My school closed years ago. There are few diploma schools available now.

I am retired now at age 71. I worked full time until I was 69 years old. Nursing is and will always be a big part of me. In my later years in nursing I felt I was often a mentor to the young, less experienced nurses. Somebody was there for me in my early years and I benefited from their wisdom and then it was my turn to pay it forward.

One of my biggest concerns is the education now being given to some of our future nurses. I asked some graduated nurses if they felt they had been adequately prepared for their jobs in nursing. Many new nurses responded with an overwhelming "No." They believed their program had prepared them more for success on the NCLEX-RN exam than for practice.

Some hospitals recognized this problem and developed a RN Residency program to teach novice nurses the knowledge and skills in order to practice good and safe medicine. They found this was needed after a large number of new graduates were leaving due to confidence and competency issues. These programs require at least a year of mentored supervision and support. Sound theories are taught as well as how to apply that knowledge and be able to make the kind of decisions needed to practice competent nursing. Critical decision making is one place some new nurses are complaining about not being prepared.

Nurses who were first LPNs told me they received more hands-on experience in procedures in their LPN school than in the RN schooling. Many newly graduated and licensed RNs have never inserted a urethral catheter or an intravenous catheter on a real patient.

The licensure exam is a minimum standard and only tests for minimum safe competency. We owe our public more. Competencies include clinical judgment and critical thinking. No amount of teaching can provide a nurse with all that's needed to know, but after the fundamentals, all nurses need to develop a spirit of inquiry and continue their education in this ever-changing and growing profession.

Good schools are trying to do the best in educating but there are schools charging a lot of money and delivering poor education. I wonder what some students are paying for today. I was told by students that there were often few explanations and fewer demonstrations and they were left to fend for themselves. Read it, get it, or find out from someone else. What happened to teaching it first?

Most new nurses don't even know what they don't know. It takes experience to be able to assess and apply clinical knowledge that produces critical thinking. Good nurses are learning every day in their practice and because they care about their patients; they ask questions of those who they feel are knowledgeable so they can learn and hopefully practice better medicine. Most doctors are willing to teach or explain something if asked and they believe you are trying to be a better nurse.

Older and experienced nurses are working with these new nurses every day. I am ashamed to say it but often that's when the "bullying" begins, and it can start when someone has an exaggerated concept of their own worth. Instead of an environment where respect and dignity should take precedence, the very lack of this is occurring. Good care relies on a harmonious and collaborative environment.

This is wrong! This situation creates major health and safety risks. It can cause increased medical errors, poor patient satisfaction, adverse outcomes, higher costs, and loss of qualified staff. There has to be zero tolerance for this behavior. But the "bullying" comes to the workplace from senior nurses, charge nurses, nurse managers, and physicians; therefore, many are reluctant to report it. The statement "Nurses eat their young" is not specific enough. New graduates are usually the group often targeted and vulnerable but they are not the only victims.

You can help, if you witness an episode of bullying, by asking that individual to help you in a task you are performing, and by also speaking up for that person. It is good to know that bystanders usually outnumber bullies.

Okay, I might as well attack the subject of "Bad Nurse" now. Every profession has them— bad doctors, bad paramedics, bad firemen, bad policemen, and of course, bad nurses. Remember, all those professions are involved in saving lives. What then makes them bad? Is it a bad education, little experience, poor circumstances, and low pay? I guess you can say that these do play a part in producing the "badness." Without a good education and training, your skills are limited. Less experience proves to lower your abilities and judgment. Poor circumstances affect our environment and can influence our feelings and attitude. And finally low pay keeps us questioning our worth.

However, I see in the good ones a belief, a belief that we can make a difference, a belief that these are God's children and that we are here to help them. It is this belief that runs through our veins, and is continually seen in our actions. We believe we are advocates, protectors, and lifelines. This commitment is burned into the hearts of the good ones.

A good nurse will continue to seek the education and experience needed to care for their patients. We, the more experienced nurses, need to "have their back" and share our knowledge with them until they feel more secure. It's the right thing to do.

CHAPTER 2

The Broken Healthcare System

What happened to health care in America? It's not the same and many don't understand how it has changed and how the changes have affected all of us.

As an experienced nurse I could see changes happening in the healthcare field—changes that were not making things better or easier for not only the patients we served, but for us, as professionals.

Here is some very important information that should be shared.

On October 1, 2013 the health insurance exchanges of the Affordable Care Act began. It has been confusing to most and now it changes the rules, as it is the law. It changes it for doctors, nurses, hospitals, and patients. Some view the changes to be good and some are totally against it. Americans have been mostly confused, and are now beginning to find out what it means for them personally.

There have been great birth pains with the startup of the Affordable Care Act, some very serious. The system is complex and confusing and there is a need to educate the public about insurance. Many staffing centers were needed to answer questions and assist persons. There have been administrative problems and more are expected but this has the potential of providing and reshaping a big part of the delivery and payment of health care in America.

There is a major problem with insurance coverage for working individuals and families. Insurance coverage is expensive and deductibles so high that many feel like they have no coverage. Employee also state that their pay has not been increasing to help with the average deductibles of $1,000 to $5,000. The deductible must be paid before there is any coverage from their insurance. Many tell me they don't go to the doctor now or have testing done unless it is absolutely necessary. There are health saving accounts, which do help, but it is still money taken from their pay.

Money continues to be the driving force for so many decisions in our world, and health care is no exception.

Medicaid is a very important health insurance for more than one-fifth of the U.S. population. The Affordable Care Act did expand coverage to millions.

In June of 2012 the Supreme Court gave the states the choice of not expanding Medicaid. North Carolina was one of those states. The state returned what I understood to be $20 million in federal funds, given to North Carolina to help establish a health insurance exchange.

Medicaid is governed under federal guidelines but each state has been allowed to set its own eligibility standards and decide which services are covered and for how long. They also decide on payment for those services, so

Medicaid policies vary from state to state.

In the *New England Journal of Medicine*, an article written by J. Oberlander and K. Perreira, and published in December 2013 on "Implementing Obama Care in a Red State," stated that the decision caused an estimated 319,000 uninsured North Carolinians to be ineligible for Medicaid even though a person's annual income was below the federal poverty level ($11,490). It stated that they were also NOT eligible for subsidized coverage in the North Carolina exchange, which left them with NO new affordable insurance options.

North Carolina is not alone; 34 states decided not to establish their own insurance exchanges, and 25 are not expanding Medicaid. Even though states rejected Medicaid expansion, some of their residents are still eligible under the Affordable Care Act (ACA) for coverage in the exchanges, but since the state has not participated in the insurance exchange, it has been left to some social service agencies to help them. The article again explained that these low income people are also ineligible for subsidized coverage in that state's exchange; therefore, many are too poor to even qualify for financial assistance to obtain insurance. The article also stated that a higher number of un-insured patients will now be seen by hospitals, doctors, and clinics, with this being a problem. The insured help to balance the financial reduc-tions in the Federal Medicare payments.

A nonprofit group called "Enroll America" is working to promote the ACA in the states that didn't decide on doing their own exchanges, and are helping uninsured persons by connect-ing them to needed resources. Some states have even tried to prevent any group from helping due to their political agenda.

If the ACA is to benefit us all, it will depend on many factors. At this time, there remain many unanswered questions. The future of health care in America is not clear at this time. It is evi-dent that money, greed, and personal interest are the driving forces and will answer many of the questions and influence the outcome. This certainly speaks to our failures in America.

It has been reported that up to 50 percent of physicians do not accept new Medicaid patients. There are many understandable reasons not to accept these patients, such as low payments, many problems obtaining authorizations for necessary tests and procedures, and difficulty getting specialty care for those who need it. It requires more time and effort by an overburdened office staff.

Some doctors don't accept Medicare either, because the payments are also low, and these payments continue to decrease for both doctors and hospitals. We hear the daily news that Medicare is going broke. It certainly worries the elderly who like their Medicare.

Other doctors have chosen to practice concierge medicine, where a person is charged an annual fee, usually $2,000 or more, along with their own insurance plan, and the person receives personalized care which includes 24-7 phone access to the doctor, no waiting in the office, possibly home care visits if needed, and many other benefits. Plans differ and one needs to check what is offered before choosing a plan. Many agree these plans are only for the rich.

Now you can get online and reach a doctor. You can ask a medical question and after paying a fee receive an answer immediately. These online doctors are available in many different fields of medicine too.

I do want to bring to your attention the Hippocratic Oath that physicians are asked to accept. It states there is to be no discrimination or interference in caring for patients due to age, creed, nationality, disease, gender, political affiliation, race, sexual orientation, ethnic origin, or social standing. I wonder and ask, what about money?

Some doctors in America are going broke and there are many reasons. Shrinking insurance reimbursements, changing regulations, drug and business costs are causing closures of many independent practices. A private practice is a small business and the payment for services is coming from insurance.

Doctors are leaving their private practices and allowing them to be bought out by hospitals. Their operating cost and not being able to negotiate better payments from insurance companies have driven them to this end. Most of us think physicians make a lot of money. Some do but new physicians struggle, due to the cost of their education. They have very high student loans and need to make enough money to not only pay these loans but run a business and enjoy a life. I don't envy them as most serve us well and they deserve good compensation.

By 2017, doctors who treat and receive Medicare payments will be rewarded or penalized in a grading system called the PVBM, or the Physician Value-Based Payment Modifier. It is based on quality and cost. Many physicians express that the concept is good but it is flawed in many aspects and cannot accurately measure any doctor's total value. The Affordable Care Act is seeking better health care for all but everyone needs to participate in the work to achieve the goals, and the ACA needs to allow all participants a voice and input into how to do this effectively.

Some have reported that at least 20 percent of Medicare patients who were hospitalized need some type of care after being discharged from the hospital. This could be from home health care with skilled nursing care, an inpatient rehab facility, or long-term hospital care. Medicare costs on post-acute care have increased without evidence of improved patient outcomes in the last decade. The president has called for changes to Medicare's post-acute payment in the 2014 budget.

Under Medicare Inpatient Prospective Payment System (IPPS) there are adjustments in payments for increased readmissions in the acute care hospitals. They are being penalized financially. The hospitals are trying to prevent readmission because they may not get paid for that readmission.

In the Congressional Research Service, some researchers said the high readmissions may be due to a number of reasons, such as poor patient compliance, inadequate follow–up of post-acute care, insufficient reliance on family caregivers, deterioration of the patient's condition, and medical errors. Many are working on how to solve this problem. It is a problem for all of us.

Poor patient compliance may be due to poor education and inadequate teaching done by healthcare personal. Failures in follow-up may be due to poor judgment of those making that decision or due to money issues of where the follow-up care is given.

Home care nurses tell me that the patients they are seeing now were discharged from the hospital earlier than in the past and their needs due to that status are much greater. Medicaid and Medicare have strict guidelines on what are approved visits by home care nurses. For example, a patient must be mostly homebound for any visit to be approved and have skilled needs.

Physicians are stating that when they need certain tests or x-rays in order to determine whether a patient has a suspected problem, Medicaid many times will not approve them.

The physician may have to send the patient to the emergency department in order to have the test or x-ray approved.

Not having someone to help care for patients after they get home is often the reason patients are sent back to the hospital. The need for home caregivers is always a problem. Families need to work and often cannot be there to provide the care some patients need. Some patients will decide to stay in their home, safe or not.

Sending patients home too early, making wrong decisions on post-care settings, and medical errors are just some of the recipes for increased readmissions and/or possible early deaths.

You need to know about health care today. It is changing and will continue to change in America. I don't have the big solutions, but I do know there are some guidelines to help you survive it.

CHAPTER 3

Today's Problems

Where to even start is a problem. Just ask anyone about their health insurance and you'll find
a problem. It is one of the biggest social and
economic problems facing America today. The
impact it has on individuals' lives is astronomi-
cal. There are many underinsured who struggle
to pay their healthcare bills. Due to the higher
healthcare premiums, deductibles, and co-pays,
increased limits on services, and having to pay
more out-of-pocket expenses, many people are
not receiving needed medical services.

In a study by the Commonwealth Fund in
2012, the underinsured were often the same as
the uninsured, namely they don't visit doctors,
don't fill prescriptions, and don't get preventive

checkups, and still many are unable to pay for the medical care they do get. It was estimated that 75 million people reported they had a hard time paying their bills even with health insurance. Healthcare benefits are a major factor in choosing a job. For those 65 and older who have Medicare (which only covers 80 percent), the cost of supplemental insurance to cover the other 20 percent can be very costly and a problem for low income retirees.

Americans will agree that healthcare reforms are needed.

America's healthcare cost is the highest of any developed country with no improvements in outcomes. Prescription medication prices due to patent protection are sometimes double what other countries pay. It has been shown in many studies the need for patients, especially with chronic diseases, to get involved in their own care. In today's changing delivery of health care, I feel this is the MOST important thing one can do for themselves and their loved ones.

Let's talk about some of the problems for

hospitals. Not only are they trying to survive, but they need to make a profit in order to expand. The American College of Healthcare Executives has reported on some of the top issues confronting hospitals in 2013. Of course, financial concerns were ranked number one. Government mandates and healthcare reforms deal mostly with reimbursements but trying to maintain patient safety and deliver quality care has its challenges and its cost.

The ACHE did a survey with hospital CEOs, and those who participated listed their concerns by order of importance. Government funding cuts and Medicaid and Medicare reimbursements rank the highest. CMS audits and the implementation of ICD-10 were also among the highest, followed by CMS and state regulations and other government scrutiny mandates. Bad debts, increasing costs for staff and supplies, reduced or delayed commercial and managed care payments, decreased inpatient volume, and competition from other providers were some others.

Safety and quality issues have their own areas of cost. The list included compliance with accrediting organizations, computerized physician order entry, staffing by trained personnel, and managing high-risk neonatal conditions, medication errors, and nosocomial infections.

If you want to read the whole report, look up the ACHE report on "Top Issues Confronting Hospitals: 2013."

I bring this to your attention as hospitals have their financial issues, and you, the consumer, are a big player in this arena. You need to understand they want your business but at the least amount of cost to them.

CHAPTER 4

Our Tech World

I need to address our tech world as it relates to today's health care. The first thing you need to know. It is here to stay. We now all live in that world; it is in our personal lives, in our businesses, and in our health care. We love our computers and we hate them.

Let's examine the effect technology has on our healthcare system. In 2009, the American Recovery and Reinvestment Act was introduced, and as of January 1, 2014, all healthcare providers were to adopt and demonstrate "meaningful use" of electric medical records (EMR) in order to be able to maintain the same reimbursement levels of Medicare and Medicaid.

This Act also included financial benefits to

those who proved meaningful use of the comprehensive history on patients, called EHR (emergency health records). The meaningful use of EHR was defined by Health IT.gov. It was to consist of using digital medical and health records to achieve certain goals:

To improve quality, safety, efficiency, and reduce health disparities, engage patients and family, improve care coordination, and population and public health, and to maintain privacy and security of patient information.

They state and hope that ultimately with compliance, it will result in better clinical outcomes, improved population health outcomes, increased transparency and efficiency, empowered individuals, and produce more robust research data on health systems.

There are penalties for non-compliance. If eligible professionals did not implement EMR/ EHR by 2015, there would be a 1 percent reduction in Medicare payment, and increased reductions are possible annually.

Because of all this, hospitals and physicians

have implemented new electronic medical record systems.

Problems with technology are not new to any of us. We've seen it in other areas of automation. You might remember when an automatic throttle system, supposed to keep a jetliner at the right speed for landing, failed and caused it to crash. It was at the San Francisco International Airport, and reported in the *Los Angeles Times*, in July 2013.

Serious problems have been reported in the past with new systems being implemented in hospitals too. The California Nurses Association press release of 7/11/13 states that there were over 100 reports submitted by RNs at Alta Bates Summit Medical Center facilities in Berkeley and Oakland. They said there were a variety of serious problems with the new system, known as Epic. A few problems cited then were: insulin orders set erroneously by the software; an inability to accurately chart specific patient needs or conditions because of pre-determined responses by computer software; lab tests not done in a timely manner; discrepancies between the Epic computers and the computers that dispense medications, causing errors with medication labels and delays in administering medications; and a nurse unable to obtain needed blood for a medical emergency.

In many states, major problems were being reported, like orders passed to the wrong patient, patients given medication they were allergic to, and in one Chicago hospital, in 2011, a patient died as a result of a massive overdose of an intravenous solution of sodium chloride prepared by an automated machine.

Many nurses and other professionals complain about the time required to interact with computer systems. It takes away from the needed time with their patients. I am very concerned about any program which prevents nurses from accurately charting specific patients' conditions because of pre-determined responses by computer software. Critical thinking is absolutely necessary to good nursing.

The next time you visit someone in the

hospital, look at what lines the hallways outside patients' rooms: multiple computers on wheels, because everyone, down to the housekeeping staff, needs to chart on these computers.

The healthcare industry is going through huge changes with government regulations and is in need of many revisions. It is evolving, and we the people are caught in this evolution. We have to be diligent and be an active participant in this system to be safe. Accountability for one-self and your loved ones is now very needed. You can reduce the chance of possible errors if you are educated in your own health issues. I don't believe the system or anyone else is out to harm you. Stay alert, knowledgeable, and active. There are wonderful, dedicated health-care providers trying to fix the problems. Each of them has a responsibility to you, and most nurses and physicians are also caught up in these same problems while they are frustrated in trying to deliver their best care to you.

CHAPTER 5

Who's Leaving Health Care

ABC News ran an article November 13, 2012 by Nisha Nathan, MD stating that by 2025 the U.S. will need 52,000 more family doctors to keep up with the increasingly older U.S. population under a new study.

The article stated that the problem isn't too few doctors in general, but according to the Association of American Medical Colleges (AAMC), too few are choosing to be a primary care doctor. The number of medical graduates who want to be in family medicine has declined by nearly 27 percent—from 5,746 in 2002 to 4,210 in 2007.

Dr. Lee Green, chair of Family Medicine at the University of Alberta, who was not involved in the study, stated, "It's tough to convince medical students to go into primary care." He added that he believes they are not well paid, treated, or respected compared to the specialists.

Many experts claim the gap between doctors and those needing care with the new health reforms will not close quickly in many areas of the country. The shortage is now in impoverished inner cities and rural areas. Some say it will get worse for some before it hopefully gets better.

There is also the nursing shortage to consider. America's need for nursing care over the next 20 years is expected to increase dramatically. The population of those 65 and older will double from 2000 to 2030. The Bureau of Labor Statistics ranks nursing occupation in the seventh highest projected job growth in the U.S., but with the increased demand for health care, the number of nurses is projected to fall by 20 percent below the need.

There are many reasons for the decline, and it has been occurring since World War II. Some are: fewer applications to nursing schools, greater opportunities for women in other, more profitable professions, shortage of nursing educators, and the aging of the present nursing workforce. The average age of a nurse nationally is 43 years old. Half of the RNs working will reach retirement age in 15 years. The average age of a graduating RN is 31, thus offering fewer years to work.

CHAPTER **6**

Good Patient and Difficult Patient

In the *New England Journal of Medicine,* Louise Aronson MD on August 29, 2013 wrote an article entitled, "'Good' Patients and 'Difficult' Patients—Rethinking Our Definitions." She describes helping her father four weeks after his heart surgery, which included a valve repair, a bladder infection, heart failure, pacemaker and feeding tube insertions, and pharyngeal trauma.

She wrote while she was assisting him off the toilet, her 75-year-old father's legs gave way and his blood pressure dropped. He was taken to the E.D. and treated with fluids. His blood INR, which is an indication of a problem with blood clotting and increased bleeding, was elevated. He was placed on monitors to check his blood pressure and alarms sounded. Nurses silenced them and increased his fluids, which helped temporarily to increase his blood pressure. But it continued to drop and his physician daughter pressed the call button and finally asked the nurse to call the doctor.

When no doctor arrived, Dr. Aronson went to the nurses' station and there "made my case" as she called it to the assembled doctors and nurses. She said they were polite, but felt their unspoken message was one of working hard, that her father wasn't their only patient, and they had appropriately prioritized their tasks. These were her written words.

She had been the caregiver and daughter, not the doctor, for her father and found some relief in leaving the doctoring to others. She said she didn't want to be that type of family member who medical teams complain about. BUT BECAUSE SHE ALSO WAS A DOCTOR AND NOT JUST A DAUGHTER, SHE KNEW SOMETHING WAS WRONG.

Acting now like a doctor/daughter instead of

a daughter/doctor, she, with the consent of her father, did a rectal exam and found blood on her gloved finger, which she proceeded to carry to the nurses' station. When the nurse returned with her to her father's room, her mother was then holding a bedpan overflowing with blood and clots. THEN, help was summoned and treatment given.

I couldn't help thinking as I read this how right she was in being the advocate for her father. Nurses and doctors often do not like the "difficult" patients or families who may question or challenge the treatment or workup. Some like to be in charge and feel others are not capable of evaluating the whole picture as they don't have the medical knowledge. There are patients and families who are certainly challenging—some mentally ill, others just high maintenance. It can be difficult dealing with them. But there are so many who make a real effort to manage their health issues, and they need our patience and deserve our attention.

In today's healthcare arena, patients and

families need to be advocates for themselves and their loved ones. I find too many not taking responsibilities for their own care and relying too much on the system, which I am here to tell you is showing signs of being in trouble. It will take collaborative efforts of all of us to success-fully and safely manage through this broken health care.

My hat's off to Dr. Louise Aronson. It was a great article. She wrote it to bring all our at-tention not only to the labeling of patients and families, but the real need for all of us to be ad-vocates, whether we be doctor, nurse, patient, or family.

CHAPTER 7

It's a Fragmented System

I want to address a big problem in the health care system: It became fragmented.

Remember when your family doctor FOLLOWED you and took care of you in the hospital? This was the person who really knew you and your health issues. And you knew them and trusted them. Not anymore. It is my belief that when the family physician was removed from the hospital bedside, it was by far the biggest mistake made in health care. It fragmented everything.

Today, we have hospitalists, doctors who don't know you but now treat you while you are in their assigned hospital. They may get some of your medical health records, if you have been in their hospital system, but so much of the time, they know nothing about you except what you or your family can tell them. Knowledge of your medical history is critical in your care. This is where part of the problem exists. The EMR (Emergency Medical Records) are supposed to help correct this, if we ever have it universally. Many physicians state it is too expensive, causes them to decrease their patient load, and even with it, there are still many reported problems.

Since the hospitalist is presented with your particular problem at the time they are treating you, they treat the problem that is causing you to be in their hospital. For many with multiple health problems, you need to understand that only the existing problem at the time of this admission is their major concern, as they then will refer you back to your family doctor for your other health issues. This can be troublesome as one health issue is often related to others.

Patients are discharged and many find themselves facing another health crisis before they can get an appointment with their family doctor, and often a readmission to the hospital is needed. Your family doctor was able to treat you totally because he had the information about all your health problems.

The hospital wants you treated but there is always an underlying concern of the cost to them, so they want you treated and discharged, as more days usually cost them more money.

Your medication may be switched to a less expensive drug for the hospital but within the same drug action family, for example, cholesterol meds. It could be one that for some reason, you are not able to take. You didn't put it on your allergy list because you didn't consider it an allergy med, but this particular one does cause you some problems.

You have the right to refuse to take any med you do not want for whatever reason. If the nurses don't agree with you, they will talk with the doctor. Hopefully you or your family know your meds and can make those decisions with good medical reasons.

If you don't know your meds and the reason

you are taking them, then find out. Know their generic and trade names, when you started taking them, and why. Make sure you have listed allergy meds, the allergic reaction you had with the drug, and those you just were not able to take for some reason, and that includes herbs and over-the-counter meds.

I'm trying to tell you why you MUST learn EVERYTHING about your own health issues. If you don't know, then start educating yourself now. First, ask your doctor and get your health records. Look up all diagnoses that relate to you. Be sure you use only good websites such as WebMD, Mayo Clinic, Cleveland Clinic, and please learn about your own health. Learn about the usual treatments for your problems and what you need to do to improve or manage them. It won't be perfect, and may be confusing, but better to have some knowledge than none. Ask your family doctor to help you.

Make and keep a written record of your medical problems, surgeries, and medications on a separate sheet of paper to be given to those who ask for it. Write dates of when a health problem began and when resolved, and who treated you and where. Mark down dates of surgeries, including the name of the surgeons and hospitals.

If you give out a copy, make sure they give you the copy back so you always have it with you.

In this book the chapter on Medical History will help you know what the hospitalist needs in order to best treat you. It was written by a very good and caring hospitalist.

YOU MUST BE RESPONSIBLE FOR YOU FIRST

Ask questions of anyone treating you. Ask why a test or lab is ordered. What are they looking for? Would the results change anything in your treatment? If so, how, and have them explain this to you.

Don't ever let a doctor intimidate you for asking questions, and if he or she tries—leave that doctor and seek another one. Don't ever be afraid to get a second opinion. Always be respectful though.

Always stay with your family in the hospital—if something doesn't sound right, STOP—ASK—make sure you question any procedures or tests until you are sure you understand and agree with them. Most people know when something is not right. They will feel it and are often too afraid to follow their instincts. Remember that hospitalist doctors do not know you or your family.

Find out if the same meds you came in on will be the same meds you will be sent home on, and if not, why? Don't be afraid to ask questions. Many mistakes are made at discharge with medications.

If you need post hospital care, home care, a nursing home, rehab, any physical or occupational treatments, then the same applies. You need to understand the reason why you need this care, and the goals that are to be achieved for you or for your family member. Then make sure there is a plan in place for success and everyone understands it. Ask if this is the only and the best plan at this time or whether another is possible.

Finding a nursing home for your loved one is a

job by itself. There is much information available on the best ways to go about this. I recommend http://www.medicare.gov/nhcompare/home.asp. Read all you can before deciding on any home. It is often one of the most difficult decisions you will ever have to make for your loved one. You want it to be the right one.

Assisted living is another area where you need to do your homework. These facilities are expensive and vary in quality and safety. The site consumer reports.org on assisted living facilities is a good place to start. The site http://www. itcombudsman.org will help you find more information and protection on nursing homes.

Remember, everyone can make a mistake, even you, so you need to be watchful.

Medical errors do happen and you need to stay alert. Meds given to you may look different, being from a different drug company. The nurse should read your wristband, ask your birthday, and tell you each med you are receiving every time. Make sure you understand what and why you are getting them. Check the information on your wristband—spelling and allergies—to be sure they are right.

Infection rates are a real problem in hospitals. To guard against infection, have anyone who touches you, including those who visit you, wash their hands first.

Hands sanitizers are usually available in each room. If something doesn't seem right, don't ignore it, ask.

All these words apply to your family members too, and that includes those who are not capable of caring for themselves. If you are their loved one, or caregiver, then you are their advocate, their voice, and you must do everything to protect them.

Get familiar with end-of-life questions, the living will, then make sure you tell your loved ones or those you have chosen to make these decisions for you (very important) when and whether you want to be placed on machines if needed and when you may not want certain procedures done. Read the medical history chapter in this book about what the hospitalist asks you to do, and follow it.

You are responsible for this. It is your LIFELINE! Believe me.

Make sure that when you (or your family member) have been discharged from the hospital that you have been given clear information and instructions on medication, purpose and side effects, and when and where you are to have follow-up care.

I recently had back surgery and I did my homework to find the doctor I wanted and the hospital. Fortunately, with my insurance I was able to choose both. If you can, you need to do this. No site's information is perfect but I think it's worth your investment. The site http://www.hospitalsafetyscore.org is a place you can look up the hospital you are considering and check out its ratings on many levels. John James, who at one time was the chief toxicologist for NASA in Houston, founded Patient Safety America, an organization to help educate people about hospital risks. He did a comprehensive study on those who in part may have died from medical errors in hospitals. He had a particular interest and then dedicated his life to improving hospital safety after his 19-year-old son died from a series of mistakes at two Texas hospitals.

Consumer Reports has published "Your Hospital Survival Guide." It contains great advice and everyone needs to read it.

Here are a few things I would also recommend when you are a patient. I had a rather complicated back surgery that required a four-day hospital stay. I was in a good hospital and had a good neurosurgeon but still there are a few things I would like to comment about. Today many hospitals, and the one I was in, required you to call in your meals to the kitchen. My daughter stayed with me the first and second day and night and my good friend stayed the next two days and nights. I highly recommend this with the surgery I had, or any major surgery. Even minor admissions need someone with them, to help if possible, and certainly those with multiple and possibly complicated health problems.

I found it difficult to even reach up to my

bedside stand to get a drink of water, turn over, or call for any food order. I knew the nursing staff would help me, when they were free to do so. I also knew there were other patients who needed them. Remember, I am a nurse and I have been that nurse trying to take care of everyone's needs, and whether others realize it, there are always too many needs and too little time. So believe me when I tell you, I loved it when family or friends were there to help me.

Stay with your loved ones if possible.

Seek legal advice if you have been in some medical harm in a hospital. There are some people today looking for any reason to sue, and it hurts all of us who need to bring attention to serious charges. Ask the advice of a trusted care doctor. Medical malpractice is often hard to prove.

Consider telling your story on the Safe Patient Project website, where advocates use these experiences to push for safer laws and regulation changes.

I hope the information given in this book will help to give you some protection.

CHAPTER 8

Medical History

I asked a practicing hospitalist what informa-tion he would need to provide the best care to anyone admitted to a hospital under his care.

Here are his recommendations in an ascend-ing order of importance according to what he feels a hospitalist needs in order to make the per-son's hospital stay as safe and smooth as possible.

1. Allergies and past medicine side effects, if any
2. Names and doses of all their prescrip-tions and over-the-counter medica-tions that they are currently taking and whether any of them have been recently changed, added, or deleted

3. Name of their primary care physician/NP/ or PA and if possible contact information

4. Names and specialty of all the specialist physicians who they have seen in the last three to five years

5. Current list of their active diagnosis and medical issues

6. List of the surgeries and significant medical procedures they have had

7. Whether they want CPR, counter shocks, intubation, and/or mechanical ventilation if needed

8. Who their Health Care Power of Attorney is and how to reach them

9. Who is their primary family/friend contact to whom information should be relayed

10. Location and approximate dates of recent hospitalizations

11. Smoking status and when started, average packs/day and for how long

12. Honest alcohol history

13. Honest illicit substance (drug) use history

14. Work, toxic exposure, and recent travel history
15. Pertinent family history
16. Diet intolerances or preferences, and if applicable, modifications, examples—pureed or thickened liquids
17. Any medical fears like needle phobia, claustrophobia, etc.

Please review this list, write the information down, and keep a copy in your papers at home; give a copy to your children, primary care physician, healthcare POA, and finally keep a copy on you, in case of an accident.

This hospitalist practices in a large metropolitan trauma center and I thank him for providing this list for all of us. He believes in providing the best care, and needs each person to help him do so.

CHAPTER 9

A Family Physician's Views

A wonderful and long-practicing family doctor expressed some concerns to me, and I do appreciate his sharing.

He had much to say about today's practice of medicine. It has also changed for him. I am sure he was able to explain or at least bring to our attention the concerns of many other physicians.

I hope it will help us to have a better understanding of some of the problems physicians face today. The following are his comments:

I am a 62-year-old physician who was in the military during the Vietnam era. Subsequent to returning home from overseas, I returned to school, attended medical school, and began practicing primary care medicine in the arena of family practice and obstetrics. My family was blue collar, and I was taught a good work ethic. I always believed that the harder you worked, the more you achieved. I've never been given financial support from my family or friends. All I have achieved is from the efforts of my wife and me, in conjunction with love from my extended family and children.

When I graduated from medical school, I owed more than $250,000 in an era where interest was over 16 percent. I was not eligible for any programs to offset those loans. Physicians and hospitals, at that time, did not generally forgive or pay off debt as part of an incentive for work, so I opened my own practice and started from scratch. I recall seeing seven patients my first day after advertising in the local community, and thinking I would never get out of debt, but I was happy to be working for myself. My practice was located in an area of need. It was generally blue collar and low income, but there were no other physicians located nearby. Essentially, I had no competition, and my practice prospered.

In the initial few years, I was on staff at five hospitals. I delivered babies at three of them, and saw all my own patients at each. There were no hospitalists back then. If I had a patient on a respirator, I managed him. If I had a patient in the NICU or CICU, a premature baby, or a 90-year-old MI patient, I managed them. I delivered babies both vaginally and by C-section, took out tonsils and appendixes, reduced dislocations, and set and casted fractures. I removed skin lesions, lipomas, and breast masses. I was the epitome of a general practitioner. There is a difference in how general or family medicine was practiced, even then, based on my location in the mountains of Colorado as compared to the larger metropolitan areas of the east. I do not believe that many practitioners of my like are, or were, available in the far east of the US.

Please don't get me wrong. I always had good specialists to rely upon when I requested, and I requested often. They were very happy to come to my assistance, and relied upon me to provide appropriate patients to them. Professional courtesy was common, and physicians in a community all knew one another. A specialist was not just a voice on the phone. We knew each other well.

I have taught students at the medical school and in a residency setting and I've had students from every level of medical care rotate through my office. I have been involved in the education process for medical assistants, x-ray technicians, ultrasound technicians, physical therapists, social workers, psychology students, high school students, foreign exchange students, nurses, nurse practitioners, midwives, medical students, residents, and physicians requiring or requesting additional experience. None of this was for reimbursement or financial gain. It was expected in the medical community that we who were established would contribute in this manner. My, how things have changed.

There have been considerable changes in the

practice of medicine over the past 35 years. Such things as legal issues; expectation of patients, employees, insurers, and hospitals; changes in technology; and many other factors have contributed to a significantly different environment today than when I first started in medicine. We all have heard our parents, grandparents, and older coworkers lament about how difficult things were, or alternatively, how great things were in the "good old days." I believe that there have been changes for both good and ill in medicine during the past generation or two, but in the end, I would not recommend that my grandson enter medicine. I shall try and elaborate fairly on both sides of the issue.

First, let's address education. An obvious difference is in the technology available now versus 35 years ago. In the 1970s, there were books and libraries. We had to buy numerous expensive texts and study them, or go to the medical library and find the books and journals we needed. In many instances, the materials were not available simply because another student had gotten to the desired material first. There were no computer resources, laptops, iPhones, or associated apps that make our life much easier now. We carried Merck manuals and other reference materials with us, and learned to use the PDR regularly. It was time consuming. We couldn't enter a key word and have the information pop up for us.

Memory was the essential key to learning and practicing, and you couldn't memorize what you hadn't been exposed to. Everything was hands-on. We learned by seeing, feeling, and smelling, and our education was deficient in that if we didn't experience it, we often didn't learn or remember it. With time and experience, we learned so much, of course, but today, students, residents, and physicians have a world of knowledge at their fingertips. Symptoms can be typed into an algorithm or data base and a differential diagnosis can almost magically appear. A diagnosis for a disease we may have never been exposed to can be entered into our iPhone and a complete explanation with treatment modalities is readily available. I don't believe that it is reasonable to suggest that learning the old way was superior to what we have today. It was different, and perhaps some might argue that it was more difficult or even better because of *how* we learned it, but I believe the current technology makes me a better physician, and that medical students and residents are better for it. I could never have imagined doing a virtual surgery, or finding instant drug cross-reactions in my phone app when I was a student.

When I was a resident, it was expected that we would work many more hours than are allowed today. We worked until the job was done, and were at the beck and call of more senior residents. It was competitive, sometimes petty and vindictive, and we made mistakes. I know many physicians and administrators who believe residents should work longer hours in order to be better practitioners. I believe this to be incorrect. We made too many mistakes when we were tired. There should be limits on the expectations of our students. Personally, I believe that it is much more an economic decision for a hospital or residency program than it is concern for the student learning. Free labor isn't given up easily.

On the other hand, the concept of entitlement seems to be growing in medical students and residents. It seems to be more about the money and benefits than contribution to community. I haven't met a single resident in the past ten years who plans to open a practice and start from scratch in a location of need. During interviews for hiring, residents seem to focus on unrealistic expectations such as high salary, rapid advances in income, excessive time off, short hours with little on-call time, payment of their loans, becoming a partner with full benefits within a short time, IRAs, etc. I don't fault someone for getting the most from a given situation, but what happened to earning what you are asking for? It took me decades to get to the position I am in now. Yes, I am considered successful in my earnings for family practice in the United States, but it came because I learned how to run a business, and I worked my ass off. I studied business, ran my own prior to becoming a physician, and I worked full time during medical school to support my family. Why should I give 50 percent of that away to someone a year after they finish their residency for essentially no recompense?

It drives me crazy when a graduating resident says, "You have a great practice that I want to take over" or "I only want to work four days per week, take two months off per year, and not do call" or "I know your practice brings in X amount of dollars per year, but I can't afford to buy in, and I expect a partnership in a year..." It also bothers me when they want to change the way I've successfully done business for years, or tell my PAs how to practice when they have 25 years' experience more than the newly graduated resident. Attitude and entitlement are issues that should be addressed in the residency. Perhaps some of my colleagues are correct in that if we don't expect a lot in residency, we can't expect a lot when they graduate.

Another great concern for me is that residencies do not teach the "business" of practicing medicine. New physicians have no concept of why we should use certain codes for billing, or how to interpret an insurance contract, or how to do the day-to-day running of a medical practice. I don't care how good a doctor you are... If you cannot run a business, you will fail unless someone teaches you or you work for an entity like Kaiser. Unfortunately, the characteristics for making a good physician are not necessarily the same as those that make a good businessman. The residencies should help their physician trainees to determine the setting where they will be most successful, and teach the basics of business for those who plan to go into private practice.

Another important issue under the heading of education is the problem of CME, or continuing medical education for physicians. I am expected to get 50 hours of CME annually to remain a member of my medical society, and most states require about the same to maintain state licensure.

Early in my career, it was easy to get appropriate CME credit. Pharmaceutical companies provided much of our opportunity to remain current in our knowledge base, and often did so in ways that were enjoyable. It was quite common to go for a weekend conference where specialists in a certain field would spend a morning educating us on all aspects of a disease state, and then we would be given the opportunity to do some other activity such as golf. Dinners with speakers who were all allowed to speak about their own research and lunch with respected specialists from university programs were common. We were able to learn about the current concepts and treatments modalities as well as the studies which were both complete and underway. Pharmaceutical companies also sponsored other CME opportunities that would go as long as a week. The sponsorship they provided allowed a discounted and reasonable fee for my attendance. I almost always tripled the 50-hour requirement every year in my early career, but now it is much more difficult to get appropriate CME.

Politicians, in their wisdom, convinced many, including young physicians, that pharmaceutical companies had an agenda of selling their products that superseded their philanthropic endeavors of educating us. I spent an hour thinking of a suitable word to use here and came up with DUH! Of course the pharm companies are trying to sell a product, but by educating me and keeping my knowledge base current, I was in a much better position to determine whether a particular product was right for me and my patients. How can it be that every other profession is allowed to be influenced by salespersons, including lobbyists for our politicians, but I, as a physician, am somehow too easily influenced? It is amazing to me how many medical communities, societies, etc. have bought into the idea that we should ethically refrain from being influenced by companies that have played such a large role in our ongoing education in the past, and that receiving anything, such as a pen with a logo, should be inappropriate and illegal. The consequence is that drug companies no longer sponsor significant CME opportunities, and the knowledge base of physicians in the community has stagnated.

Another consequence is that it is much more difficult to get samples to give to patients. In a blue collar/indigent patient population like mine, samples have always been critical. It is appalling to realize just how little today's physicians learn after they have entered practice. I used to receive five or six journals per day. Now I receive one if I'm lucky, and I make an effort to remain on the mailing lists. Teaching residents and medical students has forced me to remain current to a certain extent; however, when I talk with other caregivers in my specialty, I find many with a critical lack of knowledge in areas that I consider important. I don't mean to imply that I am better or smarter than my colleagues. I'm sure that most of the family physicians out there are smarter than me, but if we are going to have educated physicians, we better do a better job at providing opportunities.

There have been many changes in the

medico-legal field since I began practice. There has always been a target on physicians' backs when it comes to someone wanting to make some money, and defensive medicine has therefore been a way of life for all of us. I have traveled the world and found that the US is the ONLY country where malpractice is addressed in a manner that someone who is employed, receiving state or federal assistance, has filed multiple lawsuits for falls in malls, car accidents, and medical malpractice can receive 100 million dollars in a settlement for something as unprovable as loss of sexual desire (true case). A few years ago, several very large corporations were put out of business by lawsuits regarding the damage done by silicone breast implants. Now, years later, after extensive research, guess what we use in breast implants? That's right... silicone.

The cost of medicine will never come down until we have significant tort reform, but with a large majority of our legislators being attorneys, I don't expect reform to come soon. So...

the cost of medicine will remain high and physicians will continue to do many, many unnecessary high cost tests and referrals to specialists for purposes of CYA. I believe a person should always be compensated for poor medical care, but as long as winning a lawsuit is looked at in the same manner as winning the lottery instead of compensation for a tragedy, we will continue to have a problem in the system. A person who can never earn a million dollars in a lifetime's work should not be getting a 100-million-dollar settlement for any reason. We all have to pay significantly for that and our health system cannot handle those costs.

Malpractice liability has driven physicians to change or move their practices as the costs fluctuate state to state. The current attitude toward malpractice lawsuits requires defensive medicine as stated above; however, commercial insurance carriers, Medicare, and Medicaid require an ever more stringent documentation of need for labs, studies, and procedures. They say that they aren't practicing medicine and that the physician is responsible even if care is denied. For example, Medicare allows a carotid ultrasound if a patient HAS carotid atherosclerosis, but it doesn't allow the ultrasound to determine IF the patient has the diagnosis. I cannot do iron studies to determine IF a patient is anemic, but it is allowed if the patient HAS the diagnosis. Insurers are, more and more, denying studies to find out what a patient's diagnosis is. How in the heck are we to determine medicine and to perhaps limit churning and fraud, but again, tort reform is superior to these kinds of limits. We should be finding and preventing, and not waiting until the disease manifests significantly.

There has developed a significant adversity between insurers, including the government, and physicians. Medicare mandates that fraud be looked for, and insurers hire outside companies to come into medical offices to audit for overpayments. These companies are paid a percentage of the overpayments they find. Do you suppose they will offer a suggestion or two, look at the overall chart, and perhaps even help the physician in their documentation? The answer is, of course, no. Every discrepancy or deviation from what the auditor believes is a proper billing is documented for the insurer, who in turn demands repayment for not just that instance, but a projected set of similar charges over a period of years. The auditor then is paid a portion of the recovered fee. This sets up a huge adversarial situation which prevents insurers and physicians from working together. Insurers see in black and white. The government sees the patient and even the physician as a number in the computer. Unfortunately, medicine is in many subtle shades of color and there is more than one way to accomplish a goal. Ideally, that goal should be better health for all.

It has gotten more and more difficult to work with government and commercial insurers over the years, and this is one of the main reasons that I do not go into schools and recommend medicine as a career any longer. A nationalized health care without tort reform is not something I look forward to.

Other legal issues that have changed for the worse during my career include the following:

1. The legal requirement for physicians to provide various language translators, subscriptions, and language resources as well as having educational materials in multiple languages, and the ability to translate correspondence. My office has multiple persons who speak Spanish, and we otherwise have staff who speak five other languages, but I cannot bear the cost of other language services for which insurers fail to reimburse.

2. Excessive provider time is now required to do extensive documentation in all aspects of patient care to prevent auditing penalties or assessments. Charting for a purpose of providing continuing care has given way to charting to meet the varied and ever-changing bureaucratic insurance and government requirements. Additional staff time is needed to

process volumes of chart materials for those audits. Administrative paperwork to comply with state and federal regulations is staggering.

3. New legal requirements to purchase high cost electronic medical record systems which significantly reduce productivity. I do not plan to change over to an EMR system for many reasons besides cost. Systems go down, software gets corrupted, support is often unavailable or at least not timely, and productivity is reduced by half. I currently see 25-30 patients per day. That is simply not possible with an EMR in a primary setting. Most primary care physicians in my community who are using EMRs are able to see 15 at most. Finally, I do not want to sit with my back to a patient typing into a computer. I want to sit there and talk, listen, look, and feel. EMRs are not conductive to a Dr. Welby approach to medicine. If you don't know who Dr. Welby is, then I suggest you

Google the old TV show. My ideal has always been the Dr. Welby approach, but it is, in my opinion, a lost art. EMRs will be standard someday, but are impractical and unworkable for primary care in my setting at this time. Let me write my notes. I'll compare my medical care and ability to extract information with any young MD who uses an EMR. I'll score better on patient satisfaction surveys.

4. Significantly more OSHA requirements and ADA (American Disabilities Act) requirements. I am in a medical building that is clean, safe, and neat, and it has been here for 60 years. My practice is the only one in our community, but in order to update, I need to tear down the whole building and start over with permits. I have installed ramps and handicapped-accessible restrooms, yet in a recent audit it was determined that I needed to install a specialized water faucet that will never be used.

5. HIPPA (privacy act) is another set of regulations that were not in place when I came into practice. Although the idea sounds good, the practical application is absurd. How many times have you received the mandatory HIPPA form at your doctor or dentist, and thrown it away? It's as useless as a flight attendant telling me how to put on my seatbelt every time I get on an aircraft. It has kept me from obtaining critical, timely information on patients; however, it has also required that I allow a patient to request amending information in their chart at a later date.

6. Adoption of the new ICD-10 coding process will financially stress many practices. This coding is a completely new and expanded method of evaluating medical diagnoses. These extensive changes will require changes in office procedures and billing. For older physicians, this is a new thought process and will require retraining.

I could go on for some time regarding problems with insurers. It is extremely frustrating to try to understand the ever-changing requirements of each insurer. Many insurers have multiple products with no way for providers and patients to get adequate and timely information. When I was younger, we billed the patient, and it was his responsibility to deal with the insurer. The insurer did not want to lose the business of their insured and it was much easier to get problems resolved. It could not be an adversarial relationship or the insurer would lose business. State insurance commissioners would also take action in situations calling for intervention, whereas now they are not very helpful. We now spend an excessive amount of time and additional staff educating patients about their insurance plans, processing correct network referrals and formularies, and assisting them in getting their claims paid. This, of course, is all at my expense and is entirely a non-reimbursable but expensive service we provide.

There is an incredible amount of time and

effort required to work with the patients who are in most need and may be on entitlement or government programs such as Medicare, Medicaid, SSA, short- or long-term disability, new FMLA documents that every employer interprets differently, low income housing paperwork, government-sponsored utilities, court-ordered or social services-ordered documentation, phone services for after-hour services to patients, and many more similar issues. Insurers and patients do not want to pay for our time, but call and ask for advice from your plumber or try calling an attorney on the phone. I guarantee that you will be ignored or billed for the time. Somehow, it appears to be okay to call me at 3:00 a.m. to ask for a refill on your prescription or call at 5:30 p.m. to get an antibiotic so that office copay can be avoided. I am of the old school, and tend to respond to my patients anyway, but newer physicians resent and refuse many of these requests.

This leads us into more of the social/technological changes that have occurred during my career and have significantly affected the way I practice, and the way newer physicians address medical care today.

Many older physicians grew up in a time without the Internet, smartphones, or even computers. Younger physicians cannot imagine practicing medicine without these technologies, but I am concerned that there is less personalized care, less empathy, less touch and handholding. I have seen a disturbing number of instances where newer physicians are unable to diagnosis and treat without an inordinate number of labs, x-rays, and the ever-present computer diagnostic aid or iPhone application. What happened to look, feel, and touch to make the diagnosis instead of relying on a multitude of expensive tests and a computer? The idea of treating over the Internet by messaging or emails, without an office visit, is foreign to me, and once again raises the questions of liability and reimbursing me for my time.

By not embracing these new tools, patients are beginning to complain that they should be entitled to see their medical records online, make appointments, obtain care and advice based on labs or other information they email from outside sources, or have their prescriptions immediately processed electronically. The importance of face-to-face care is being trivialized. I understand these modalities are not wrong, and will certainly become commonplace; however, older physicians often do not understand the technology or outright refuse to do so. I am reluctant to institute electronic medical records as stated previously. I refuse to type into a computer when I believe I should be looking at my patient as they speak to me. I also refuse the cost, the hassle factor, the legal implications, and the reduction in my ability to see the number of patients needing to be seen. I will not halve the patients for twice the cost. Newer physicians do not have the luxury to have my attitude. The newer technologies are being forced upon us at lightning speed. Certainly, they will be standard in the future, but the transition is very difficult for us dinosaurs, and a more flexible implementation time would be helpful and, I believe, more successful. Ironically, younger physicians will face many similar issues by the time they are closer to retirement. I have heard that 90 percent of what our total human knowledge base will be in 50 years will be discovered during those 50 years, and I believe that will continue to cause huge changes in the social and technological aspects of medical care.

A very frightening aspect of the new social media technology is the ability of a patient to adversely affect or destroy a physician's reputation by posting angry, negative, and oftentimes untrue accusations. If a patient wants narcotics, specialized testing, medications, referrals, work or school excuses, handicapped placards, jury duty excuses, unfounded disability diagnosis tests and does not receive what he or she wishes, they can write any derogatory remarks they want and post it as an opinion, thereby negating the ability for the physician to have it removed or to successfully file slander charges.

Physicians fear bad publicity and often comply with an individual's request against the patient's or public's best interest to make that patient happy, and avoid or diminish both overt and covert threats. Most patients do not seek out medical evaluation websites to write positive reviews. Those who do take the time generally do so if they are angry. Many physicians I know have countered this by hiring companies to flood the sites with good evaluations, thereby burying the angry, vindictive reviews. I believe that this tactic is understandable but unethical si I have occasionally asked several of my long-term patients to write a review. The bottom line is that the system is flawed and skewed. The idea of a patient being able to peruse reviews on a physician is good, but in reality, it doesn't work.

One of the saddest changes I have witnessed in the past several years is the increasing intensity of patient demands, patient feelings of entitlement, and their associated dissatisfaction, which often results in patient abuse of staff and providers. I have been stabbed, hit, had things thrown at me, and threatened with bodily harm and even death on multiple occasions. Virtually a day never goes by where at least one patient is upset when asked to provide an insurance card, fill out insurance-required paperwork, and wait while insurance is verified or pay required co-pay. If a patient is told their insurance has terminated and they are now self-pay, somehow it is always the staff's fault. Many times the patient will then expect payment to be waived. There is an increased lack of responsibility from many patients. They expect the provider to be knowledgeable and accountable for their insurance needs. They forget that the responsibility for meeting their insurer's criteria for coverage is on their shoulders.

I'm not sure how new physicians will handle these ever-growing problems, but my solution is to ask the patient to leave and escort them to the door. I have had to occasionally call the police for support. It is unbelievable to me how common courtesy has given way to intolerance and the personal belief of entitlement over the past several years. Is our society now so fast-paced that any delay in gratification justifies the rudeness that is so prevalent today? I expect a two-year-old to demand instant gratification and have a self-centered attitude. Unfortunately, many persons of all age groups are acting like two-year-olds.

At the risk of overstating this problem, I must say that the current acceptance of poor attitude and behavior is very sad. When people start believing that medicine is a right and that I—or any person, from physician to store clerk—am there to satisfy their every need or wish, intolerance and abuse become commonplace. Call me old-fashioned, but I don't believe that medical care is a right. It is something that must be earned and paid for, if not by the patient, then by society; even when care is given, it does not mean that every need can or should be met.

The young physician who wishes to open a private practice must now also become an expert in Human Resources. With the new or additional employee state and federal employment requirements and regulations, one must be an attorney, negotiator, psychologist, financial planner, and the go-to person for all of the staff needs. Many hours are needed to maintain a staff that is dedicated and loyal.

With more of our population becoming covered by state and federal programs, we can expect even more controls and limitations. The idea of rationing is already being implemented in some states. It will be difficult for patients to understand and accept these changes. I believe that age and diagnosis will determine who gets what care, and tighter controls will be placed on testing, medications, and treatment plans. Medical professionals who are trained to do their very best for their patients will struggle with these decisions. Many older physicians are already making the decision to retire early.

As I read over these long notes, I realize that there are many challenges facing older as well as younger physicians. The challenges appear to be increasing. I look back over the years and know that I could never have been in any other profession. I have laughed and cried and experienced the most joyful times and the most painful times. It is not possible to just throw out a life vest to a drowning patient. One must get into the water, muddy and torturous, and swim, struggle, and pray. In the end I hope that others will say of me, "He really did so much, he cared so much, and we will miss him."

CHAPTER 10

Hospice

I need here to write about hospice and my experience working there. When people hear the word "hospice" they think death. Once a woman told me, "You go in on a cart and come out in a box." I can tell you this isn't always true, but there is so much more to tell.

Hospice comes at a time for many when it seems all hope has left them. They face a situation where their physical health is now being questioned and this affects their mental health. The mere fact that someone has suggested hospice, for many, is explosive, with many different reactions following.

I worked as an admission nurse. Referrals were called into our facility when a doctor or family felt hospice services could benefit a person. A time was set up and we would then meet with the person and family to see if hospice was not only appropriate but if they wanted our services. Those places were homes, hospitals, and nursing homes.

Every situation is different. There are some families that welcome us and have had some experience with hospice in the past and understand what we have to offer. They are ready, physically and mentally, and very little explanation is required. Services are started with everyone agreeable and satisfied.

Then other times we need to explain what hospice's philosophy is and what it can mean to those who might be eligible for its services. It is never easy to talk when a person's life is being questioned. We know about living but we don't know about dying. Haven't we all questioned our dying? What will be the cause? When will it occur? Will there be suffering? Some have had some experience, when an illness brought them closer to death. Just trying to live becomes a challenge. I've heard my patients say, "I am tired of being tired." That old saying "It's not how long you live but how well you live" comes into play. I have seen mothers, suffering much, who have small children who would do anything for one more moment with them. You see, it is all so personal and individualized. That is how it needs to be handled. The person leads the way. We listen to them, their wants, their needs, and then do our best to provide the care to match those wants and needs.

Hospice isn't perfect. It is made up of people, and people aren't perfect. But I did see hospice educate those who worked for them about their philosophy and how to present it. They offered many ongoing educational programs to help the workers do the best job in the field. Sometimes it just doesn't work out for some for so many reasons, but for most, I can tell you, they were glad hospice was there for them.

Hospice was some of the most rewarding work I've ever done. To help people at a time when they are facing a crisis, to be with them, each person left me with an understanding of how I personally want to handle my own end-of-life issues. It may not be death we fear but dying, and I'll choose hospice to help me.

CHAPTER 11

The Minimum List

In some areas in America, the EMS systems ask people to put their printed health information in a plastic container on the shelf in the refrigerator and mark the container with a red marker "health info" so it can be easily seen by the paramedic. If they have a signed DNR (do not resuscitate) paper it should also be in that container.

You need to carry with you at all times a minimum list. Carry it in your purse or wallet. The bigger information can be left at home. Just make sure your loved ones know where to find it.

Here is the list to carry at all times:

1. Name, address, home phone number, and emergency contacts' phone numbers—more than one please
2. Insurance information
3. Primary doctor or nurse practitioner with address and phone numbers
4. List of active medical diagnoses, medical problems, surgeries, or treatments
5. List all medications, names, doses, when taken, and include over-the-counter medication and herbs
6. List all medication you cannot take, allergies or side effects

CHAPTER 12

Final Words

Many believe America has changed and that we are now a greedier nation. Has respect declined and selfishness increased? Is there a "ME" generation? Politicians are rich, and getting richer. Some don't seem to care about what is really good for America; they care about getting re-elected and keeping that status. Rules, laws, policies, and government mandates are often made without realizing their true consequences. Many realize there are problems, because they or their loved ones, in some way, have suffered from them.

It is up to you to do everything to protect yourselves and your loved ones.

Andy Rooney could say so much with so few words. Here are a few quotes I really like.

I've learned…That we should be glad God doesn't give us everything we ask for.

I've learned…That to ignore the facts does not change them.

I've learned…That sometimes a person needs a hand to hold and a heart to understand.

I've learned…That I can always pray for someone when I don't have the strength to help him in some other way.

I've learned…That it's those small daily happenings that make life so spectacular.

I've learned…That when you harbor bitterness, happiness will dock elsewhere.

I've learned…That everyone you meet deserves to be greeted with a smile.

I've learned…That love, not time, heals all wounds.

I've learned…That the best classroom in the world is at the feet of an elderly person.

I've learned…That when you're newly born

grandchild holds your little finger in his fist, you're hooked for life.

I've learned…That you should never say no to a gift from a child.

I've learned…That under everyone's hard shell is someone who wants to be appreciated and loved.

I've learned…That when you're in love, it shows.

I've learned…That just one person saying to me, "You've made my day!" makes my day.

There are more but these express some of the wonder and truth for all of us.

Be good to each other, all of you, whether you are working in the medical field or not. I know that each one of you is a unique child of God. I've spent my whole life believing in that philosophy. I've tried to be the best advocate for my all my patients and pray that each one of you will do the same for yourself and family. Therefore, any interaction we have with each other should always be based on love. May God bless and watch over us all.

www.ingramcontent.com/pod-product-compliance
Lightning Source LLC
Chambersburg PA
CBHW072335290526
45794CB00002B/883

* 9 7 8 1 4 7 8 7 8 0 7 1 7 *